PROVEN NATURAL REMEDIES FOR COLDS, FLU and COLD SORES

Difference Between Colds and Flu Symptoms
Prevention Treatment and conventional Therapy
Prevention and Treatment and Natural Therapy
Difference between Flu and Bird Flu symptoms
Causes of colds and influenza
Cold Sore is general Known as Herpes Simplex

Dr. Arta Tran Dash, M.Sc., M. S., Ph. D.
Retired Professor

INTRODUCTION

PROVEN NATURAL REMEDIES FOR COLDS, FLU and COLD SORES

What are Common Colds and Flu (influenza)?

Although you may get cold any time of the year, normally flu seasons start from late fall through the winter, they are caused by any of more than two hundred viruses, but most common ones are rhinoviruses, that infect the upper respiratory tract.

Difference between Colds and Flu

It is important to know the difference between the two. The difference mostly lies in severity and duration of the condition. There are over 100 viruses that can cause common colds, but these two viruses rhinoviruses and coronaviruses usually cause common colds. Common cold affects the upper respiratory tract (nose and throat.) It is considered only a minor viral infection of the nose and throat.,

Cold symptoms normally last for about a week. During the first three days that you have cold symptoms, you are contagious. This means you can pass the cold to others, so stay home and get plenty of much-needed rest.

Where as, flu (commonly used for influenza) is caused solely by the viruses namely type A and type B of the three influenza viruses; type A, B and C. accompanying initially by symptoms, such as chill, high fever, aches and pains followed by severe cough, sore throat, and fatigue. These viruses enter the body through the mouth, nose, and eyes. For detail symptoms see below/

A bout of flu normally lasts **one to two weeks**, with severe symptoms subsiding in **two to three days**. However, weakness, fatigue, dry cough, and a reduced ability to exercise may continue for **three to seven days**.

Most healthy adults become contagious the day before symptoms develop (which makes it trickier to prevent from spreading). They remain infectious for up to five to seven days after symptoms appear. Some infected persons show no symptoms, yet can spread viruses to other persons.

Symptoms of Common Colds

- Running or stuffy nose, sore throat, cough, and in some cases mild fever
- Cold symptoms are generally milder
- Sneezing, headache
- Colds generally do not result in serious health problems

Symptoms of Flu.

Symptoms usually appear from one to four days after exposure to the virus,
General malaise accompanied by
- running nose, sneezing, and coughing;
- congestion, sore throat, and dry cough;,
- dry hacking cough, shaking chills
- fever, chills/sweats, muscle aches, and joint pains;
- fatigue and weakness
- swollen lymph glands;
- stuffy and running nose
- nausea, vomiting, and loss of appetite
- severe fatigue that may last up to two weeks;

LOKA SAMASTA SUKHINO BHABANTU

(Let Each And Every Person In The Universe Be Hale and Hearty)

VEDAS

DISCLAIMER

This book is not intended to diagnose, treat or replace the service of a doctor. If you have any health conditions or are under a doctor's care, you must consult your physician or a healthcare professional before you apply any of the recommendations set forth in the pages of this book.
All information available in this book is for educational purposes only, and none of the stated products have been FDA approved. Any application of the recommendations mentioned in this book is at the readers' discretion and sole risk.

The publication is offered "as is" without warranty of any kind either expressed or implied, including but not limited to, the implied warranties of merchantability, suitability for a particular purpose or non-infringement. Descriptions of or reference to products or publications does not imply endorsement of that product or publication.
Here is how you can use the information in this book to improve your health and wellness. Being Empowered with these powerful armies of information, and the knowledge gathered from it, you would be able to discuss your health problems with a healthcare professional and design a regimen that is conducive to your health and well being, instead of just being drugged to death and suffer from lethal side effects of these drugs, causing serious debilitating, chronic diseases, even death.

If you find your physician is unwilling to discuss the issue, find another physician or a healthcare professional who is more sensitive to your wish and willing to take the time to listen to you for your well being. You need to know all your options before embarking on a particular regimen or a procedure.

TABLE OF CONTENTS

Astragalus

Vitamin C

Elderberry extract

CHAPTER THREE

Preventions

Annual flu shot

Antiviral drugs to prevent and treat colds and flu

Tamiflu

CHAPTER FOUR

Natural alternatives

Flu vaccines

Vitamin C, ginseng

Shark liver oil

Boost your immune system

Natural supplements

Immune fortifying herb

Grandma chicken soup

Natural Supplements

Other therapeutic agents

CHAPTER ONE

PROVEN NATURAL REMEDIES FOR COLDS, FLU and COLD SORES

CHAPTER ONE

PROVEN NATURAL REMEDIES FOR COLDS, FLU and COLD SORES

What are Common Colds and Flu (influenza)?

Although you may get cold any time of the year, normally flu seasons start from late fall through the winter, they are caused by any of more than two hundred viruses, but most common ones are rhinoviruses, that infect the upper respiratory tract.

Difference between Colds and Flu

It is important to know the difference between the two. The difference mostly lies in severity and duration of the condition. There are over 100 viruses that can cause common colds, but these two viruses rhinoviruses and coronaviruses usually cause common colds. Common cold affects the upper respiratory tract (nose and throat.) It is considered only a minor viral infection of the nose and throat.,

Cold symptoms normally last for about a week. During the first three days that you have cold symptoms, you are contagious. This means you can pass the cold to others, so stay home and get plenty of much-needed rest.

Where as, flu (commonly used for influenza) is caused solely by the viruses namely type A and type B of the three influenza viruses; type A, B and C. accompanying initially by symptoms, such as chill, high fever, aches and pains followed by severe cough, sore throat, and fatigue. These viruses enter the body through the mouth, nose, and eyes. For detail symptoms see below/

A bout of flu normally lasts **one to two weeks**, with severe symptoms subsiding in **two to three days**. However, weakness, fatigue, dry cough, and a reduced ability to exercise may continue for **three to seven days**.

Most healthy adults become contagious the day before symptoms develop (which makes it trickier to prevent from spreading). They remain infectious for up to five to seven days after symptoms appear. Some infected persons show no symptoms, yet can spread viruses to other persons.

Symptoms of Common Colds

- Running or stuffy nose, sore throat, cough, and in some cases mild fever
- Cold symptoms are generally milder
- Sneezing, headache
- Colds generally do not result in serious health problems

Symptoms of Flu.

Symptoms usually appear from one to four days after exposure to the virus,
General malaise accompanied by
- running nose, sneezing, and coughing;
- congestion, sore throat, and dry cough;,
- dry hacking cough, shaking chills
- fever, chills/sweats, muscle aches, and joint pains;
- fatigue and weakness
- swollen lymph glands;
- stuffy and running nose
- nausea, vomiting, and loss of appetite
- severe fatigue that may last up to two weeks;

How Does Cold and Flu Spread?

Colds and flu spread mostly by coming in contact with contaminated objects and infected individuals. Furthermore, the cold and flu viruses can survive on objects like pens, books, coffee mugs, door knobs or any other contaminated objects for several hours, which can infect individuals who come in contact with them. In addition when sneezing and coughing become air borne, the persons nearby are in high risk of being infected. Thus, it is easy to come in contact with the viruses during daily life.

However, if your immune system is in peak form, you can fend off the cold viruses. The only way you will get cold, if you have weakened immune system. If you have a compromised immune system, you open the door not only viruses to enter your body also various other diseases.

Causes of Colds and Flu

1) Sedentary life style and improper diet are not only the most important factors for   being inflicted with colds and flu, but also for other chronic degenerative diseases.
Familiar Adage: Foods that can kill, foods that can heal.

Intake of highly processed foods, refined carbohydrates (ie., refined sugar, white bread), fried foods, coffee, alcohol, smoking. They may depressed the immune system response, making the body vulnerable to infections, and also to other degenerative diseases.
2) poor elimination, and lack of exercise
3) toxicity in the body
4) lack of sleep
5)lack of flora and flora imbalance
6) a weakened immune system due to life style factors, nutritional
   deficiencies and high stress levels.Cold, a Poorly Understood Health Conditions

Common colds and flu are overly misunderstood health complaints. A cold is not a disease. it is rather the cure of a disease. Most importantly, one should understand that the various annoying and irritating symptoms of are processes by which the body is trying to eliminate, restore, and maintain equilibrium. When the body is overwhelmed with toxins, it is working fast and furiously to find ways to flush out and re-establish internal balance. Researchers believe that body is using cold viruses as a means of detoxifying itself through mucus elimination, fever, sweats, and reduced appetites. Furthermore, they also believe that fever prevents viruses and bacteria from replicating, or in other words, fever is frying these viruses and bacteria.

Mad Rush to Local Drug Stores

Any neighbourhood drugstore carry a bewildering array of weapons to uproot the foe, the common cold—antipyretics, antihistamines, decongestants, sedatives, and many others, like acetaminophen and ibuprofen , which are also generally recommended by physicians, even in our childhood. These over-the-counter common cold drugs do not cure colds, rather mask their symptoms without regard to the underlying root cause. Furthermore, these drugs have serious side effects.

Caution: Don't give aspirin to children with flu, since it may cause Reye's `syndrome in them.

Effects of Suppressing Common Colds

As we mentioned earlier, body is desperately trying to cleanse and detoxifying itself from internal congestion and toxicity due to chronic self-poisoning. If the colds are actively suppressed, the body ultimately becomes unable to release internal toxins safely. Thus, in the long run, lead to chronic degenerative diseases, such as bronchitis, emphysema, and other serious diseases possibly heart attacks, stroke, cancer, and diabetes. The body needs external help to release internal toxins not through drugs, but by means of natural nutrients, proper diet, exercise and rest. If it is not properly looked after, it may lead to a dangerous disease called pneumonia.

CHAPTER TWO

Prevention: Natural remedy

Flu Vaccines

Flu vaccines are manufactured six months ago according to the strains at that time. But present strains are different. I don't know how the vaccines manufactured six months ago is going to be effective for the present flu strain.

However, if you do decide to take vaccines as advised by your doctor, insist that you want the vaccine from single vial, because multi vial has thimserol preservatives which contains mercury that is dangerous

Every time you come from outside into the house, always wash your hands with soap, then wash your face

Homeopathic remedy for prevention of flu.

- **Influenzinum**, potency 30 C or 200 C liquid. Take once a month. Press the top to pump twice under the tongue during the flu season only (i.e. November to April)

- **Anacoccinum** like Oscillococcinum or Oscillo, is a homeopathic remedy for flu remedy in the 200C potency. **recommended when strong flu symptoms have started to appear**. It is the preferred choice of people looking for a natural solution to beat back a sudden and harsh flu attack. **Anacoccinum** can help you recover from the flu gently and more quickly. Natural and safe. Made according to the HPUS (Homeopathic pharmacopoeia of the United States) and FDA regulations.

  Rhus Tox, dose: potency liquid 200 C/2x daily to prevent cold and flu during flu season.

  Press the too twice to pump two times under the tongue

  This is an extremely useful medicine. It not only protects you from flu, fever, typhoid, aches and pains, it is also a **pain killer**, relieves joint pains, soreness, arthritis. It is also one of the best remedy for prevention and cure of cataract, glaucoma
  Take this once a day during flu season to prevent cold and flu

- **Arnica Montana**, it is also a pain killer. Sore from workout, sports injury, aches and pain, after surgery, dose: potency liquid 3o C, just squeeze two times under the tongue. Don't take two often, only when necessary

- You can get this from any health food store or they can order for you

  These two remedies always keep at home in a cool place, use it whenever needed. They both are also pain killers

  NOTE: sometimes it is hard to get in liquid. Most places you get in pellets. Just follow the instructions in the bottles or ask the health sture. You put certain number of pellets under the tongue.

Vitamin D3: D3 is a potent antimicrobial agent producing 200 to 300 antimicrobial peptides in your body that kill bacteria, viruses, and fungi. It reduces the risk of developing flu and dying from the flu. It increases microbe killing compounds. Vitamin D3 deficiency will impair the immune system response, opening the door not only cold and flo, but also to other diseases. You know vitamin D3 is panacea. It prevents every disease, including heart attacks, cancer, strokes, diabetes, Alzheimer's, and Parkinson's, and so on. Never be deficient in vitamin D3.

Ttake 6000 IU daily, take 3000 with meal at lunch and 3000 with meal at dinner for men.

For women: 2000 IU at lunch and 2000 IU at dinner

Probiotics: or Acidophilus bifidus

Probiotics keep our immune system primed and ready to fight or combat these winter bugs. You can buy supplements or consume fermented foods like yogurt (yogurt is a healthy snack when combined with super foods like blueberries, and strawberries, it has plenty of protein and calcium,) kefir, tempeh, sauerkraut, kimichi, to nae a few.

Probiotics are absolutely required for healthy gut. Gut is not healthy nothing will be healthy. It is also required for healthy immune system response that protects against infection.

NAC: N-acetyl cystein
_Helps prevent flu
- Precursor to master antioxidant
  Glutathione which is considered life
  Helps treat chronic bronchitis
  Good for a diverse array of conditions
  Also longevity, inflammation, mood, cognition, energy
Dose: 500 mg

Astragalus: protect against **cold and flu. Boosts immune system**, anti-inflammatory, antiviral, prevents growth of tumor, reduce high blood pressure, regulates and prevents diabetes, cholesterol lowering, protects body from physical, mental and emotional stress, cancers, especially melanoma and leukemia,
This herb boosts production of white blood cells as well as the body's powerful antiviral chemicals known as interferons.

It causes your body to produce more telomeres part of your DNA that protects chromosomes from dying. It increases the rate of replication of immune cells, also increases the production of an enzyme telomerase which enables the production of more telomeres that make you live longer

Astragalus also produce more NK (Natural Killer Cells) cells in the immune system, may cause cancer cell death.

Astragalus is known for increasing the quantity and quality of sperm
Dose: 200 or 259 in the morning in empty stomach and same dose in the evening

Vitamin C: prevents cold and flu. Take 6000 mg in divided doses. It packs a powerful punch against cold and flu. There are situations when a person dying from influenza who made complete recovery with high enough IV doses of ascorbic acid (C). IV of ascorbic acid can help remission of cancer. Vitamin C is water soluble. It is difficult to over dose. For maintainance take 300 mg in divided doses. If you get cold or flu, increase the frequency of taking vitamin C , take 1000 mg every four hours. It may help reduce the severity and duration of cold and flu. It is also a good laxative in high doses.

Women should not take than 500 mg, may be a little more nut not more than 1000 mg, if they are intending to bear child or pregnant or nursing without consulting doctor.

After taking all the preventive and curative measures, if you still get flu, then follow the measures discussed below

Have **elderberry extract** at home, take it according to instruction if you get flu. This will get rid of flu and cold 2 or 3 days. **This is a powerful flu fighter.**
Also take vitamin C (1000 mg) every four hours.
Take Rhus Tox, every four hours

Lavender: lavender essential oil is calming, soothing, relaxing, and smells great. You can use it for wound treatment, relaxation and pain relief. It is gentle enough to rub directly on skin and has a soothing effect. Rubbing the oil on feet and neck of a sick person helps him sleep better and recover faster.

Stay Gydrated

Drink green tea, or rooibus tea, or chamomile tea, or ginger tea or dandelion tea, or peppermint tea, eat very light if you have to. Keep hydrated with hot water or the teas. Do not add milk to the teas mentioned above. You will lose all the benefits.

Chewing fresh ginger gives relief from sore throat, although it might have burning sensation at first.

Take chicken soup: don't buy chicken soup from stores. They are loaded with salt and other preservative chemicals. It will cause more harm than good

How to make chicken soup

-   Get chicken backs and bones around 1 lb, depending upon how much you want to make, enough to make to drink whole day

-   Put onion, garlic, ginger, cut pieces of celery, carrots, bell papers, anything else you like Put this entire ingredient in a large pot. Put enough water and salt to taste. Bring the water to boil until the Chicken is tender

    Adding fresh chopped garlic to chicken soup gives immune system a powerful boost. Garlic not only kills germ, it also appears to stimulate the release of natural killer cells, which are part of the immune system, and arsenal of germ fighters, and spike the soup with cayenne to increase the broth's decongestant power.

-   Take the soup water in a bowl with some pieces of chicken and vegetables (if You want) or just the water. Keep taking It at some intervals of your choice
    If finished, put some more water and boil.

Health Benefits of ginger

Note Women trying to get pregnant or pregnant or nursing should not take ginger

Ginger health benefits are well known:: relieves muscle pain, indigestion, upset stomach, digestive problems, etc.

However, the recent clinical studies have shown that ginger is scientifically shown to help:

* **Dissolve** deadly blood clots
* **Boost Blood Circulation** and cure vericose veins
* **Prevent Painful hemorrhoids,** increase vein health and improves healthy blood flow
* **Improve blood pressure fast** - and keep blood thin and healthy
* **Eliminate joint and muscle aches** - helping you to bend, flex and point
* **Boost energy levels to new heights** and infuse oxygen rich blood to every part of the body
* **Keep you mentally sharp** - putting an end to foggy thinking, memory loss of seniors
* **avoid a heart, brain, or lung disaster...**
* **Significant reduction in cholesterol**
* **increases the strength of heart**
    A new study has found a combination of two delicious spices ginger and chilli paper
     Cou;d slash your cancer risk
* **increase energy production in heart-** to enhance pumping within heart cells that is required

for optimal cardiac output and much more

Medical report published in *Prostaglandins Medicine* states that ginger significantly reduced cholesterol and thromboxane synthesis (a substance made by platelets that causes blood clot formation and constriction of blood vessels)

It is also reported that ginger increases heart's strength . This is is why scientists call ginger a *cardiac tonic agent* because of its ability to increase energy production in heart and to enhance punping within heart cells that is required for optimal cardiac output.

Reports published in *Thrombosis Research* have shown that ginger is an effective anti-coagulant that can literally *melt away* blood clots *which could trigger heart attacks.*

According to the *Prestigious National Institute of Health* ginger administered to coronary heart patients produced a **significant reduction** in blood platelets clumping.

Reference
Health Research Labs

How to Take ginger
there are several ways you can take it
- take skin out and grate it put in curry, you can't do that Arati have to eat.
   you can put in yours after it is done
- put it in smoothies

- you can make tea: again take the skin out. slice it, put it in a put all the slices (make enough slices) in a pot you may cut into smallpieces
  and boil it 10 - 20 minutes. drain the water out , you may also put green tea bag on it, so get many benefits of both
  A very healthy tea.
  you can cut those slices into small pieces put them on food and eat
  I also mention to take 3 or 4 cloves garlic every day. Garlic has similar properties

There are various natural and conventional remedies for cold and flu discussed below. There will be some repetitions. The purpose is to reinforce further the concept of natural healing, and compare the difference between conventional approach (which have serious side effects) and natural healing approach. .

CHAPTER THREE

Prevention and Treatment: Conventional Therapy

Preventions:

Annual Flu Shot

Flu vaccine is a sort of quick fix aimed at preventing one health danger, flu, ignoring underlying health problems. Moreover flu vaccine has serious side effects, namely it contains neurotoxins because of the mercury-based preservatives. Adverse reactions to flu vaccines range from being mild to lethal, namely reddened eyes, facial swelling, and respiratory symptoms. Even if there are no side effects, yet there is one major problem—-

flu vaccines are not 100 % effective, because flu vaccines are manufacture before the common flu strains are realized, hence they may not contain the same common strains for the ensuing flu seasons, thereby making them ineffective for protecting the flu patients, during the peak flu season.

Note: even if you have taken flu shot, you still might get flu, however, the severity and duration are substantially reduced.

If you don't want to take a flu shot, read on. There are various alternatives for protecting and preventing yourself from flu.

Antiviral Drugs To Prevent and Treat Colds & Flu

The antiviral drugs normally used to treat/prevent colds and flu are amantadine, rimantadine,oseltamivir (Tamiflu), zanamivir. These drugs are approved by US Food and Drug Administration for treatment or prevention of colds and flu.. For the last couple of years, Tamiflu has been more popular. See below.

Tamiflu

Tamiflu is an antiviral medicine, which is being heavily prescribed by the doctors during the flu season. Tamiflu belong to a group of medicines known as neuraminidase inhibitors. Tamiflu attack the flu at its source by killing the virus that causes the flu, rather than masking the symptoms; and stops spreading inside your body.

Tamiflu is usually well tolerated, however tamiflu may cause the following side effects:

- nausea,
- vomiting
- diarrhea,
- dizziness,
- headache,
- nosebleed,
- bronchitis
- eye redness or discomfort,
- sleep problems (insomnia), or
- cough or other respiratory problems.
- The flu itself or Tamiflu may rarely cause serious mental/mood changes. This may be more likely in children. Tell your doctor of any signs of unusual behaviour, including confusion, agitation, or self-injury.
- However, taking with food my abate some of these side effects.
- Contact your doctor within 48 hours of the onslaught of common colds and flu.

CHAPTER FOUR

Natural Alternatives

Flu Vaccines

As mentioned earlier, Flu vaccines are manufactured six months ago according to the strains present at that time. But present strains are different. I don't know how the vaccines manufactured six months ago are going to be effective for the present flu strain.

However, if you do decide to take vaccines as advised by your doctor, insist that you want the vaccine from single vial, because multi vial has thimserol preservatives which contains mercury that is lethal. May cause several chronic degenerative diseases, like Alzheimer's.

Wash your hands frequently, that may prevent half of all cases. Every time you come from outside into house, wash your hands with soap, and then your face.

Vitamin C is not a cure for common colds or flu, but certainly can help relieve the symptoms of colds or flu. Moreover, if it is taken regularly 1000 mg twice daily (one in AM, noon, in PM, if you have diarrhea, then just take once), it will substantially reduce the risk of having common colds or flu without any side effects Dr. Linus Pauling: **Vitamin C and Common Cold.** –

Ginseng: Recently, besides numerous other benefits, ginseng is now medically proven to be effective in the treatment of common colds and flu. It is known to have reduced the symptoms of common colds and flu. CTV or CBC news.

Shark Liver Oil
A book entitled **"Miracles Healings"** by four medical doctors, Neil Solomon, MD, Ph.D., Richard Passwater, Ph.D., Ingmemar Joelsson, MD, Ph.D., Lenard Haines discusses clinical studies relating to shark liver oil and reported their **miracle healing** for many health problems, namely
- highest immune system booster;
- allergies, asthma, and arthritis;
- inflammation in the arteries (doctors say this is the main cause of heart attacks;)
- colds, flu, and others;
- diabetes, MS, high blood pressure;
- rashes, sores, psoriasis, dermatitis, fungi, and others;
and improves general well being for all ages.

Dr. Hubert said that since his own school-age children took shark liver oil as a protection, they have no colds or flu. There are other testimonials to these effects.
Ref. Alive, 2005, Nov.277, p.75.

 wait Homeopathy: Rhus Tox, use it before flu seasons start which may help prevent getting flu. If you do get flu, the severity and duration will be lessened, and use it again to reduce the symptoms of common cold and flu. See later.   .

Boost Your Immune System

DIET

(a) Eat foods rich in cysteine, a precurser to glutathione---avocado, asparagus, broccoli, spinach, and walnuts. Recall that glutathione not only boost our immune system, but also our life depends on it. Also increase selenium levels by consuming foods, such as brewer's yeast or nutritional yeast, brazil nuts, almonds, garlic, barley, fish, especially shell fish, zinc level should also be increased by taking foods like chick peas, legumes, brewer's yeast, and deluse.

(b) **Mushrooms**: mushrooms, such as shitake, maitake, enoki, oyster, reishi are known to bolster the resistance to all sorts of stress, and extend longevity. The recent research in Japan and US has shown that maitake has important anticancer, antiviral, immune enhancing effects. It may also help reduce high blood pressure, and blood sugar. Maitake taken daily can produce general tonic effect. However, research indicates that combining different mushrooms can become more effective than only one kind. Research studies indicate that reishi mushroom can not only enhance immune function, but also has anti-inflammatory effect. It may be helpful for people with rheumatoid arthritis, and osteoarthritis. Give it a try.

See Andrew Weil, MD. Protect Your Immune System. A Look at Chinese Tonics. alive, Dec. 2005, No. 278: p.42
.

(c) Foods to Avoid
All these foods described below suppress the immune system response, thereby suppressing the production of white blood cells making the body unable to combat the viruses, and also other degenerative diseases. Thus, avoid foods---refined sugar, refined carbohydrates (white bread, white flour..), highly processed foods, processed meats (bacon, sausage, Deli), packaged foods fried foods, trans fats, hydrogenated fats, margarine, alcohol, coffee, smoking.

Note:
Consumption of sugar seriously hampers the two important cells—
Macrophages (called "pac-man" cells, devour up foreign invaders, i.e. bacteria,
Fungi, etc.), natural killer cells (NK-cells) that go after cancer cells and virus-
Infected cells. But one teaspoon of sugar can inhibit macrophages and NK-cells for
up to six hours, making you vulnerable to cancer and infectious diseases.

Natural Supplements

Vitamins B, C, complete E (tocopherols, tocotrienols), R+-alpha lipoic acid, CoQ10, grape seed extract, and glutathione. See later for details.

(e) Homeopathy: One of the most vital homeopathic remedy that enhances the immune system response is commonly known as "Thymuline 9 CH". It consists of a set of   five vials. Use one vial each per week. Take the dose under your tongue on an empty stomach for five weeks. It is an extremely diluted thymus extract that activates our immune system by overseeing the thymus gland. The thymus gland is a key part of our immune system.

(d) Immune-Fortifying Herb

(e) Ginseng:
It is proven to produce a state of improved resistance to stress, and to have helped increase our ability to combat diseases by revving up our vitality and fortifying normal bodily functions. A recent study has proven that ginseng helps relieve symptoms of common colds and flu, and increase antibodies to fight flu viruses.
Astragalus and Echinacea are known to have immune-supporting activity.
Treatments (Natural Alternatives)

(a) Recommended diets: drink mostly fluids, such as soups and broths, and herbal teas.

(b) Stay hydrated. Drink at least 8 to 10 glasses of pure water daily. This will help relieve stiffness and loosen the secretion.

(c) A traditional drink for colds and flu is prepared by boiling water with ginger, cinnamon, and bay leaves, and drain the liquid, and add fresh lemon juice, and honey to this tea. Drink the tea every two or three hours daily. This will help soothe your throat and chest, stop mucus buildup, and stimulate cleansing sweat.

(d) Grand Ma Chicken Soup: In a big pot boil organic chicken with water in a medium heat adding onion, ginger, garlic, bay leaves, cloves, cinnamon, and add salt to your taste. You may add cut pieces of carrots.. Boil them until the chicken is tender. Drink the broth every three hours. This will relieve the symptoms of colds and flu. Chicken contains high levels of amino acid cysteine that supports the mucus in the lungs and make it less sticky so that it can be secreted easily. Cysteine also helps enhance the glutathione levels which strengthens immune system along with other significant benefits.

(e) Do not take juices, especially orange juice. As you know they all contain sugar, that will inhibit the production of white blood cells which thye body needs to combat the viruses and bacteria. This means you will just prolong your suffering. Also eliminate milk and other diary products from your diet while you are sick with colds and flu, since they stimulate the production of mucus and that will only make the matter worse.

CHAPTER FIVE

Primary Recommendation

Homeopathy

(a) Sometimes a combination homeopathic cold remedy available in local health food Stores. Take them at the onset of colds and flu.

(b) Rhus Tox. This remedy effects on flu having symptoms with aches and pains in all bones, sore throats with swollen glands, sticking pain in swallowing, fever, typhoid type of fever, restlessness, trembling, chill as if cold water poured on, followed by heat, and desire to stretch to limits. See the dose instruction later.

Note: after using the homeopathic remedies, if the symptoms improve within 24 hours, stop using the remedies, start if the symptoms reoccur. However, if you don't experience any improvements within 24 hours, select the remedy that best suits your symptoms from homeopathic therapies discussed later in this chapter.

2. Take vitamin C (ascorbic acid with bioflavonoids) 1000 mg to 2000mg every two hours, as long as the bowl can tolerate during viral illness. Vitamin C revs up immune system response by increasing the production of white blood cells enhancing the body's antiviral and antibacterial activities, and enabling it to combat the viruses and bacteria. Vitamin C has antiviral, antibacterial, and antihistamine properties. Dr. Linus Pauling, in his book **"Vitamin C and the Common Cold"** reported that by taking 1 g (1000 mg) daily (only if you are over 14), it was possible to prevent common colds.

Vitamin C makes the immune system strong.

4. Take zinc 25 to 50 mg. Take elemental zinc or zinc lozenges (zinc gluconate or chelat) every two hours while awake. Take zinc only if you are over 14 years of age Zinc enhance immune system function and may have antiviral activity and also helps body utilize and maintain the level of vitamin A. Stop taking zinc this high and this frequently   for more than a week or if nausea occurs.

5.Echinacea fortifies the immune system against infection by activating both phgocytosis (the process by which the white blood cells devour up invading microorganisms) and the production of virus-killer cells of the immune system. It substantially relieve the severity of symptoms of both colds and flu and hasten the recovery process. Do not take this for a longer period.

6. Take 1 or 2 capsules of aged garlic extract (preferably aged garlic extra) every two hours until the symptoms of colds and flu are gone. Fresh raw garlic is more preferable and more effective. Eat or swallow two cloves of chopped garlic at the first sign of cold or flu. You may sprinkle chopped raw garlic in soups or salads. In addition to garlic having antiviral and antibacterial effects, it has also blood-cleansing activity. Thus, you should take garlic every day, whether you have cold or not. furthermore, taking fresh raw parsley with raw garlic can prevent "garlic breathe."

7.Shark Liver Oil : see discussions earlier.

8. Take fresh ginger tea every couple of hours. You may add cinnamon, bay leaves. To the mixture add fresh lemon juice and honey to your taste.

General Recommendation

The remedies recommended above are extremely effective for common colds and flu. Although you can use them individually, but using two or three of them in combination have been found to be highly effective. The other remedies discussed below can either replace or supplement the ones given above and may be combined when suggested doses are observed.

Antioxidants
To prevent any disease, especially infectious diseases, we must have our immune system in peak form. In order to achieve this, we must observe diet, have adequate rest, proper exercise, reduce stress, and finally have basic natural nutrients. If you take all these precautions, these will enable you to live longer and healthier.

-   high potency multiple vitamin, rich in minerals (calcium, magnesium, zinc,..;)

-   vitamin C, 1000 mg, three times daily;

-   complete vitamin E (tocopherols, and tocotrienols), 400 IU twice daily;

-   R+-alpha lipoic acid, 100 mg twice daily;

-   CoQ10, 100 mg twice daily

- Resveratrol 500 mg daily

- Grape seed extract (or pycnogenol), 300 mg twice daily;

- Omega 3 fatty acids, 1000 mg twice daily

HERBS

- **Astragalus:**
- protect against **cold and flu. Boosts immune system**, anti-inflammatory, antiviral, prevents growth of tumor, reduce high blood pressure, regulates and prevents diabetes, cholesterol lowering, protects body from physical, mental and emotional stress, cancers, especially melanoma and leukemia,

- This herb boosts production of white blood cells as well as the body's powerful antiviral chemicals known as interferon's.

- It causes your body to produce more telomeres part of your DNA that protects chromosomes from dying. It increases the rate of replication of immune cells, also increases the production of an enzyme telomerase which enables the production of more telomeres that make you live longer

- *Astragalus also produce more NK (Natural Killer Cells) cells in the immune system, may cause cancer cell death.*

- *Astragalus is known for increasing the quantity and quality of sperm*

- **Dose:** 200 or 259 in the morning in empty stomach and same dose in the evening
-
- Caution: do not use astragalus if you have a fever;
-
- Panax ginseng:

- we have mentioned earlier that it has been medically proven that it is highly effective in the treatment and prevention of common colds and flu. Ginseng is known to develop a state of resistance to stress, and our ability to resist diseases by revving up general ability and fortifying our normal bodily functions.

- Goldenseal: it is an antiviral and immune stimulant. Discontinue using it if nausea, loose stools or other gastrointestinal symptoms occur'

- Prepare a tea by infusing equal parts of three herbs, namely **Elder Flower, Yarrow,** and **Peppermint.** Take one tbsp of each of the herbs steep them in 8 oz of pure water for thirty minutes and strain. Drink the tea freely through out the day.

- You may also make in analogous manner the tea by infusing cinnamon, sage, and bay leaves.

- Geranium, unique to South Africa, is known to reduce the severity of colds, and shorten duration of colds and the upper respiratory tract infectious illness, for instance sinusitis, and bronchitis, whether it is of viral or bacterial origin..

CHAPTER SIX

Homeopathy

General Information

At the onset of colds and flu pick the remedy from this section that best parallels your symptoms and use doses of potency 6C (3 pellets) or 30C (3 pellets) by dissolving them under the tongue for every three or four hours for three days. If your conditions improve, stop taking the remedy unless the symptoms reoccur. If your condition does not improve, then select another remedy.

- Aconitum Napellus is for colds suddenly inflicted by by exposure to dry, cold whether. Other symptoms include, sudden onset of fever with chills, rapid pulse, face flushed, swollen, one chick red, the other pale, scratchy throat with thin nasal discharge, nostril swollen, anxiety, restlessness, chilly with thirst
  .

- Allium cepa is a remedy effective for colds with copious watery burning, extremely acrid nasal discharge. Conditions become worse in warm room and towards evenings, better in open air. Other symptoms include, reddened eyes with profuse tears, tingling sensation in nose, with tending to violent sneezing, and sensitive to smell of flowers.

- Antimonium tart   its therapeutic applications matches to terrible cold that lodges in the chest, rattling of mucus in the lungs that is very difficult to spit it out. Other symptoms include, weakness, drowsiness, fever with trembling, chilliness, intense heat with copious perspiration. Patients feel better in cold, open air, and worse in lying down, worse in warm room and damp whether.

- Arsenicum Allum is used in colds with stuffy nose, copious clear running watery mucus from the nose making the upper lips red. The patient feels chilly and crave for warm drinks, and feel anxious and restlessness

.

- Belladonna relieves the following symptoms: nasal discharge stops suddenly and is replaced by congestive trembling headache, sudden onslaught of high fever with hot head and cold extremities, flushed face, reddened lips and gums. . patients is very hot but not perspiring, no thirst, has a strong pounding pulse, hallucination when eyes closed and frightening dreams. The face looks flushed and red, eyes look glassy. Symptoms are more pronounced on the right side of the body.

- Gelsenium is one of the most common remedy for flu, especially when the symptoms linger even after the flu; colds withmuscle aches, patients feel drowsy and fatigued, can open the eyelids only half way, because the eyelids feel heavy, frequent sneezing and chillness in the back, a unique symptom of this remedy includes a feeling of relief after urination.

- Pulsatilla is a remedy for symptoms involving mucus membranes all affected, thick yellow-green discharge, worse at night, particularly lying down, dry mouth, but no thirst, loss of smell and taste, symptoms ever changing. A good female remedy.

- Nux Vomica is a remedy for: nose running all day and stuffed at night, feels worst in the morning, throat raw and sore, body very chilled, and the patient feels irritable. Nux helps immune system working well. It is frequently the first remedy after too much dosing, rendering a sort of equilibrium and eradicating chronic effects

Antibiotics: don't use antibiotics for colds and flu, because colds and flu are viral, whereas antibiotics are for bacterial diseases. Antibiotics don't kill viruses, so they are not effective in treating colds or flu. However, in severe cases, where a secondary bacterial infection developed, their use may be needed.

Aromatherapy

It has been proven that many essential oils have antiviral and antibacterial activity. Clinical studies have proven that inhalations of pure organic aromatic essential oils freeing the airway passages relieving congestion of common colds, so that the patient can breathe easier. This suggest that using aromatic essential oils around the house either by diffusing in the air, massaging, or using them in bath, can help disinfect the air around the house, and also make the air breathable. Furthermore, studies have shown that many essential oils have been found to possess the antiseptic, antiviral, and antibacterial activity to to combat certain strains of viruses and bacteria.

Below is a list of essential oils that will prove beneficial for not only relieving the symptoms of colds and flu, also help prevent from getting colds or flu.

Ravensara Aromatica: It is mildly cleansing, antiseptic, and strongly antiviral

Add 12 or 15 drops into a mist bottle that contains 30 ml of pure water and spray into the air inside the house to protect you and your family from airborne bacteria and viruses. Also use it as inhalation if you have cold or flu, that will relieve your congestion and help you breathe easier. Lemon (citrus limonum) is antibacterial, astringent, and cleansing.

Use two drops of Eucalyptus and 4 drops of Lemon essential oils into a diffuser and spray in the air not only to kill airborne bacteria, but also to create a clean bright fresh antibacterial environment.

Peppermint (Mantha Piperita) has a cooling and cleansing aroma, effective for head cold and sinus congestion.

If you have cold or flu, use 2 drops of peppermint and 2 drops of lemon oil into a hot water bowl. Inhale as often as you can until your congestion is cleared. Be sure to protect your eyes.

Tea Tree Oil is a strongly antiseptic, antibacterial and antiviral; effective for colds and flu. In a tub with hot water having level ½ or one inch above naval, add 12 drops of tea tree oil and a cup of Epson salt, bath for 15 minutes; keep your legs up the water.

You may elect to diffuse just tea tree oil into the air to make the air clean and fresh, free of airborne microorganisms.

Lavender (lavendula officinelia): it is the most versatile of all essential oils, and known to be an excellent relaxing and antiseptic oil.

You may combine 4-6 drops of lavender oil with all other oils mentioned above (or on its own) in a diffuser,or bath, or a message (with sesame oil, or walnut oil).

Note: if you have cold, choose a combination of essential oils that match your symptoms. Take a few drops of each on your palm, rub the palm together, inhale or smell several times until your congestion is cleared.

Reference

1. Danlelle Sade, B. Sc., Nutrition/Certified, Aromatherapist. Directions, Dec/Jan, 2004; p.9

2. David Crowe. One bad shot. Should you get a flu vaccination this season? alive, 2005, Nov. 277; pp.66-69.

3. Danlello Sade, B.Sc., Nutrition/certified Aromatherapist, *Relieve cold & Congestion.* Directions. 2004, Dec/Jan; p.9

4. Gary M Skole C.P.I., Scott Greenberg MD., Michael Gazs. **Self-Care Anywhere**. New Century Publishing, 2000'

5. Heather Caruso. B.Sc., D.H.M.S. H.D. *Homeopathy for Colds.* Directions 2004, Dec/Jan; p.22.

6. James F. Balch, M.D., Mark Stengler, N.D. **Prescription fo Natural Cures.** John Wiley & Sons, Inc. 2004.

7. Michael Downey, *Natural Alternative to Flu Shot.* Vitality Dec.2004/Jan. 2005; p.40-42.

8. Michael Murray T. Murray, ND. *If you don't a flu shot:* Natural Immune boosting. Alive, Oct. 2005; No. 276, p. 78-79.

9. Neil Solomon MD, Ph.D., Richard Passwayter,Ph.D., Ingmemar Joelsson, MD, Ph.D., Leonard Haines. **Miracle Healing: Shark Liver Oil.** *Colds & Flu* alive. 2005, Nov. 277; p. 75.

10. Nicole Duelli, CCH *Homeopathic Profile. Its sniffle Season/.* alive. 2005, No.Nov. 277; p. 60-61.

11. Dr. Pauling. **Vitamin C and the Common Cold**

12. Ross Trattler ND, with the assistance of Adrian JonesND. **Better Health Through Natural Healing.** Hinkler Books Pty Ltd.2003.

13. www.NewDirections.on.ca

14. www.BellLifestyleProducts.com

CHAPTER SEVEN

AVIAN/BIRD FLU

What is Bird Flu (Avian Influenza)?

Bird flu is an infection caused by influenza A (H5N1), subtype of the type A influenza virus. Wild migratory birds worldwide generally carry the viruses in their intestinal tracts,

But it does not make them sick. It is highly contagious and can infect domesticated birds, including chicken, ducks, and turkeys; not only make them sick, but also kill them.

How Does Bird Flu Spread?

The reason it is called Avian Flu, because wild aquatic birds are the source of influenza viruses. As we mentioned above, the viruses that live in the intestinal tract of wild waterfowl, normally does not cause the disease. These birds shed a high concentration of of influenza viruses through saliva, nasal secretion, and feces. Vulnerable birds (poultry, ducks, turkey) get infected when they come in contact with contaminated excretions or surfaces that have been contaminated with excretions. It was noted that most cases of Avian Flu infection in humans were caused from contacts with the infected poultry or contaminated surfaces.

The transmission of avian flu virus from one person to another has been known to be extremely rare, and transmission has not been reported to continue beyond one person/. Past flu pandemics were caused due to the virus having antigenetic shift from animal to human and genetically mutating into highly lethal strains capable of transmitting through air, and bodily secretions.

Note: you don't get avian flu by eating poultry or eggs if they are properly cooked. Properly cooked meat kills all the viruses. However, under cooked meat and ducks blood have been involved in H5N1 cases in Asia.

**Difference between Bird Flu Viruses and Human Influenza Viruses:
Types, Subtypes, and Strains**

There are three types of influenza viruses A, B, and C. the influenza types A, B, and C viruses can infect humans. However, influenza type A and its subtypes viruses can not only infect humans, but also can infect birds, pigs, horse, and other animals. Furthermore, wild migratory birds carry influenza type A viruses in their intestinal tracts, without getting sick.

The subtypes of flu type A viruses are classified on the basis of the combinations of surface proteins, namely Hemagluttinins, (HA) and neuraminidase (NA). There are 144 possible combinations HA and NA proteins. But in fact, some combinations have not been discovered. Scientists believe that some combinations of the subtypes can't be formed. However, this fact has not been proved. To illustrate subtypes, consider , for instance, "H3N2 virus" which typifies an influenza A subtype that has an HA 3 protein and an NA 2 protein. Analogously, H5N1 virus is a combination of HA 5 protein and NA 1 protein.

The influenza A subtypes that are currently in circulation among the people worldwide include H1N1, H1N2, and H3N2. The subtypes that are generally found in animal species include H7N7 and H3N8 viruses. These viruses cause illness in horses and H3N8 also has recently been found to infect dogs.

Difference

All known subtypes of influenza type A viruses can be found in birds.. however, when we talk about "avian/bird flu" viruses, we mean influenza A subtypes, H5N1, mainly found in birds.

Now what exactly we mean by "human flu viruses"? there are only three known subtypes of type A flu virus, namely H1N1, H1N2, and H3N2, that are currently in circulation among people worldwide. It is possible that some genetic components of current human flu type A viruses come from birds originally.

Next we discuss what are "avian/bird flu" viruses. First of all, all known subtypes of type A flu viruses can be found in birds. However, when we talk about "avian/bird flu" viruses, we mean subtypes of influenza type A virus, H5N1, mainly found in birds.

Instances of Avian Flu Infections in Humans

Influenza A subtype H5N1 virus was first isolated from birds in South Africa in 1961. like all bird flu viruses, H5N1 virus is present in birds worldwide. It is highly contagious among birds and can be extremely lethal. Although, bird flu bird flu virus H5N1 normally do not infect humans, but several instances of human infections with bird flu have been reported since 1997.

When there is an outbreaks of avian/bird flu among poultry (chicken, ducks, and turkeys), there is every likelihood of people getting infected who come in contact with infected birds or contaminated surfaces. For instance, the recent outbreak of avian influenza A, H5N1, virus among poultry in Asia and Europe led to human infections and deaths. However, ,the transmission of avian flu H5N1 virus from human to human rarely occurs. See below for a few instances of human infections and deaths.

- The avian flu H5N1 virus outbreak in Hong Kong in 1997, among the poultry spread to human infections and deaths. 18 people were infected and 6 of them died. Inorder to contain the outbreak, authorities destroyed roughly, 1.5 million chickens to eradicate the sources of the viruses. Scientists found that the avian flu virus spread mainly from poultry to human, however seldom human-to-human infection was noted.

- More recent outbreaks of avian influenza H5N1 occurred among poultry in Asian countries, namely Cambodia, China, Indonesia, Japan, Laos, South Korea, Thailand, and Vietnam during late 2003 and early 2004. During this period, more than 100 million birds have either died from infection or have been killed by the authorities to contain the outbreaks.
- Again new outbreaks of influenza H5N1 occurred among poultry around June of 2004 in Cambodia, China (Tibet), Indonesia, Kazakhastan, Malaysia, Mongolia, Russia (Siberia) Thailand, and Vietnam. It seems these outbreaks are still ongoing.

- The most recent outbreaks of influenza H5N1 among poultry in 2005 occurred in Turkey, Romania, China, and Canada (BC). In December 2005 in China brother and sister were infected with avian flu virus, the sister died, the brother survived, and also in December of

- 2005 Indonesia suffered another avuin flu outbreak,where 12 persons were infected, and eight died. . The spread of influenza H5N1 from human to human has seldom been reported., moreover, the transmission has not been documented beyond one person.

- In January 2006, roughly 14 people in Turkey were infected with H5N1 virus, although roughly 48 people were found positive to be positive with the H5N1viru. Out of 14 infected people with H5N1 virus, three children belonging to one family died. Fortunately there was no cases of human to human transmission, otherwise it would have led to pandemic creating havoc in the world. Avian flu still continuing in these countries.

Symptoms of Avian Flu in Humans

The symptoms of avian flu in humans are similar to typical influenza-like symptoms, but more severe. They range from typical flu-like symptoms (fever, cough, sore throats, nausea,, and muscle aches) to eye infections(conjunctivitis), pneumonia, viral pneumonia, acute respiratory illness and other severe and life-threatening conditions leading to death.

Prevention of Avian Flu

There is currently no avian flu vaccines available to protect humans against H5N1 virus. Scientists are attempting to develop vaccines to protect people against H5N1 virus.
In Hungary, officials proclaimed that preliminary experiments with an H5N1 vaccine declare it works. The Hungary's Health Minister and dozens of people were inoculated with the vaccine and after three weeks tests showed that the antibodies to the virus had appeared in their blood. Although the results are preliminary, he is 99.9 % sure that the vaccine works. The world Health Organization has not conformed the results.

- one other thing people could do is to take seasonal flu vaccines to protect themselves from influenza A virus. This may help develop immunity to against avian H5N1 virus.

- In order to protect yourself from avian flu in the absence H5N1 flu vaccines, antiviral drugs may help. It is proven clinically that they are effective in both preventing and treating the disease. See details later.

- The standard tests for influenza A viruses can be reliably employed to detect avian flu infections in humans.

As you know, the drugs and vaccines have serious side effects. If you do not wish to take drugs or flu vaccines, then follow the suggestions given below for safe alternatives.

Safe Alternatives

1. keep your immune system in peak form by consuming immune-boosting foods, avoiding immune-suppressing foods, reducing stress (meditate regularly), and doing exercise regularly; and taking natural nutrients. Follow the instructions given in the chapter on Colds & Flu.

2. staying informed and being informed is very crucial to protecting yourself and your family from avian flu epidemics. It is not certain that a vaccine will be developed in time to fight avian flu virus. Even if an avian flu vaccine is developed, by the time it is commercially circulated, it may be ineffective to fight the most recent strains of flu virus causing pandemics/. If pandemics occurs, it may advisable to limit your contact with the general public for an extended period, however, impossible it sounds.

3. wash your hands frequently.

4. virus spread when a person comes in contact with infected birds or contaminated surfaces, and then touches his or her eyes, nose, or mouth..\

5. avoid contact with people who are sick with virus. If you are infected, keep your distance from others to protect them getting infected. Also cover your mouth and nose while coughing and sneezing, which will protect people around you from getting infected.

Treatment

Four different types of antiviral drugs, namely armantadine,, rimantadine, oseltamivir (Tamiflu) and zanamavir are recommended FDA to treat influenza A virus in humans . All four drugs are effective against influenza A viruses. However, sometimes influenza strains can become resistant to these drugs, and render them ineffective. For instance, some of the 2004 H5N1 viruses isolated from poultry and humans in Asia have been found to be resistant to two of the antiviral drugs, namely amantadine, rimantadine. Although research relating to avian flu viruses for resistance to influenza antiviral drugs is continuing, oseltamivir, and zanamivir still seem to be effective treatment at the present time.

Tamiflu (oseltamivir): STAR ANISE

Tamiflu which is effective in reducing the symptoms of Avian Flu, though not cure or prevent it , is made from a naturally occurring herb that is grown in China during Marcjh and May .this licorice-flavoured herb is traditionally used in many of the flavourful Chinese dishes, including spare-ribs and five-spice duck. It is also used in stewed meat to enhance its flavour and is, in fact, one of the ingredient in traditional Chinese five-spice powder,, available in any Chinese grocery stores.

In Chinese medicine, star-anise has been used for the treatment of respiratory blockage which according to experts is the way which the avian flu kills its victims. Although for practitioners of Chinese medicine the natural source of tamiflu is intriguing, many Chinese think tamiflu is a Chinese herbal remedy, except it is pharmaceutically altered.

Traditional Chinese medicine practitioners place emphasis on strengthening body's immune system. Thus, if you are worried avian flu, strengthen your immune system by following suggestions described in chapter on Colds&Flu , such as taking immune enhancing foods and avoiding immune depressing foods, natural supplements, regular exercise, and reducing stress through meditation otherwise. See also Albert Nerenberg. **STAR ANISE.** Tamiflu's Main Ingredient plentiful in Chinatown. Toronto Star, Oct/ 30, 2005/

Pandemic Flu

The Avian Flu H5N1 virus normally does not infect humans, although there have been some cases of infection due to contact with infected animals (poultry, or pigs) or contaminated surfaces.

Until now, spread of H5N1 from human to human has been almost non-existent, and has not continued beyond one person. However, H5N1 virus is dynamic and continually evolving. A sudden or an abrupt radical changes occurs in influenza A viruses subtypes as a result of a process called *antigenetic shift* producing a novel influenza A virus subtypes. Antigenetic shift may take place either through animal (poultry, pig)-to human transmission or through mixing up mixing of human influenza A virus and animal influenza A virus genes to produce a new human influenza A subtype virus through a process known as *genetic reassessment.*

This new virus is created by new combinations of the HA and NA proteins on the surface of the virus. Since this novel virus is not currently in circulation in humans, there is no immune protection against it in human population. If antigenetic shift lead to the emergence of a new influenza A subtype, a global influenza pandemic may occur.

Since our immune system is totally defenceless against these pandemic viruses, which will create disaster of titanic proportions worldwide. Scientists predict, in the absence of any proper treatment and preventive therapy, up to 1 billion people could die all around the whole world.

Reference:

- Michael T. Osterholm, Director, Centre for Infectious Disease and Policy, University of Minnesota.
- Dinitry K. Lvov, Director, D. I. Ivanovsky, Institute of Virology, Russian Academy of Medical Sxiences.
- Rita Daly, MDs reveal worst-case scenario, Toronto Star, Oct. 30, 2005.

CHAPTER EIGHT

Influenza Pandemic during 20th Century

During this period of time, there were the emergence of new influenza A virus subtypes that caused three pandemics spread worldwide within one of year of detention.

- 1918-18, "Spanish Flu" [A, H1N1] caused highest number of influenza deaths around the world. More than 500,000 people died in United States, and roughly 50 million people have died worldwide. Many people died within the first few days of infection, while others died of complications later. About half of those died are young and healthy adults. Influenza A (H1N1) viruses are still in circulation today after being introduced again into the human population in 1977.

- 1957-58 "Avian Flu" [A, (H2N2)], led to roughly 70,000 deaths in United States. The virus was first detected in China in late February 1957, spread to US by June 1957.

- 1968-69, "Hong Kong Flu" [A, (H3N2)], led to around 34,000 deaths in US. The virus was first isolated in Hong Kong in early 1968 and spread to US later that year. Influenza A subtypes H3N2 viruses still circulates among humans today.

  Both the 1957-58 and 1968-69 pandemics were the result of viruses containing combination of genes from a human influenza virus A and an avian influenza A virus subtypes. The origin of the 1918-19 pandemic viruses is not known.

Prevention and Treatment of Pandemics

- The most important factor in preventing pandemic is to keep your immune system in peak form, so that the body will be able to defend itself against the viruses. Follow the instructions discussed earlier for prevention.

- Antiviral medications amantadine, rimantadine, oseltamivir, (Tamiflu), zanamivir are approved by FDA for the treatment or prevention of influenza A viruses. All four work for influenza virus. However, some of these drugs may not always be effective, because influenza virus strains can become resistant to one or more of these medications. For instance, the influenza A subtypes H5N1 viruses are resistant to amantadine, rimantadine. Although, monitoring of avian flu viruses for resistance to antiviral drugs is still continuing, oseltamivir (Tamiflu) and zanamivir appear to be effective treatment for influenza viruses at the present time.

  o However, most recent cases in Vietnam (December, 2005), where four people infected with avian flu virus were treated with Tamiflu, all four died. Tamiflu was ineffective in all these four cases. Most likely the avian influenza virus mutated to new virus strains that became resistant to Tamiflu. If this happens during pandemic, it will spell disaster and consequences will be unpredictable and uncontrollable.

  o US and Canada, probably other countries are amassing millions of doses of Tamiflu in case pandemic occurs. However, according to an article in Wall Street Journal, Oct. 11, 2005, and the above incidence in Vietnam, there are signs that avian flu viruses are already mutating making hem resistant to Tamiflu. Moreover, if every body is using Tamiflu for seasonal flu, there is every likelihood of influenza strains developing increased immunity to it. If this happens, pandemic flu will create unstoppable havoc. .

- Shark Liver Oil, many other natural nutrients and herbs discussed in Colds and Flu Section might greatly reduce the risk of getting infected with avian flu,

- Currently no vaccine is available for the emerging strains of avian flu. Once a potent pandemic strains of influenza virus is isolated, it will take several months before a viable vaccine is commercially available. If a pandemic occurs, probably most countries are unprepared, including United States.

-

Preparing For the Next Pandemic

Many scientists worldwide surmise that it is only a matter of time before the next influenza pandemic arrive with vengeance. The severity of the next pandemic disaster is unpredictable. Scientists and MDs around Toronto predict when next pandemic disaster strikes Toronto, more than 900,000 people will fall ill, and more than five thousand may die. Imagine how many millions will be infected in whole of Canada. Modelling studies indicate that effects of influenza pandemic in the United States could be disastrous, both in terms of human deaths and financial hardships.

In the absence of control measures (i.e. vaccines and drugs)), it has been estimated that in the United States with a full-fledged pandemic could create havoc, infect any where between 15 % to 35 % of US population, and economic impact could range between $71.3 166.5 billions. Imagine the severity of pandemic that could create havoc both in terms of human deaths and financial disaster

.

In the event of pandemic and absence of control measures, doctors, nurses ambulance attendants, and hospital workers will be in state of fits and helplessness as they encounter exodus of flu-stricken patients cram the emergency departments. Hospitals will cancel non-emergency surgery and redeploy all their resources to meet the demand of this unpredictable event. Hospital administrators will also be forced to adopt what is called "battlefront triage" as doctors have to make heart-rending decisions on which patients to save and which one to let die.

This is a very difficult situation for healthcare professionals to let people die unattended, contradictory to the very philosophy they have taken oath for. As the death toll mounts, morgues, crematoriums, and funeral homes will be crammed and overflow, refrigerated trucks will serve as temporary morgues. Also retired doctors, nurses, and healthcare professionals will be asked to help out. Thus, take enough precautions following the suggestions given in Chapter on Colds and Flu both in terms of prevention and treatment.

Reference
Michael T. Osterholm, Director, Centre for Infectious Disease Research and Policy at the University of Minnesota.
Dinitry K. Lvov, Director, D. I. Ivanovsky, Institute of Virology, Russian Academy of Medical Sciences
Albert Nerenberg, Tamiflu's main ingredient plentiful in Chinatown : STAR ANISE/ Toronto Star, October 30, 2005.
Rita Daly, MDs reveal worst-case scenario. Toronto Star, October 30, 2005.
www.readyforcrisis.com

CHAPTER NINE

COLD SORES

(Herpes Simplex Virus)

Cold Sores and Symptoms

Cold sores, also called fever blisters, are small but painful fluid filled blisters, usually found on or around the mouth, lips, and nose, including gums and conjuctiva. They have been known to be caused by temperature changes as the name suggests "Cold Sores" , in fact , however, they are caused by one of two highly contagious herpes simplex viruses type 1 (HSV1) and type 2 (HSV2).

Herpes simplex virus type 1 produce oral herpes or cold sores, where as type 2 causes genital herpes infecting genital tracts. Both type 1 and type 2 viruses can infect oral tissues. However, more than 95 % of cold sore outbreaks are caused by type 1 virus. The viruses lie dormant in roughly 09 % of people.

The causative factors that activate and replicate the viruses are:
- stress and anxiety
- diet
- tenperature changes
- sexual contacts
- weakened immune system
- nutritional deficiencies
- local irritation and other illnesses

Symptoms

- local irritation, itchy, tingling sensation, tenderness, accompanied by mild fever as well as swollen lymph nodes in the neck, with one or more clusters of small painful pus-filled blisters

Herpes (cold sores) affects the nerve cells of the spinal chord (genital herpes) and the nerves at the base of the brain (oral herpes). The virus is highly contagious, even more so when liquid filled blisters are present. Thus, any person infected with oral or genital herpes must not let these affected areas come into direct contact with another person. Once the herpes simplex virus types 1 and 2 have been transmitted, the infection is permanent, that is, the viruses don't leave the body. They can remain dormant in nervous system for life.

An outbreak is commonly accompanied by flu-like symptoms with tingling, tenderness, and itching in the areas where the eruptions often trigger cold sore blisters, mostly occur on lips, throat, mouth (oral herpes). Thus, tingling, itchy, areas becomes a few small pus-filled blisters. These blisters ruptures or ulcerate and scab over. These lesions are highly contagious until crusted over.

During this phase any area of broken skins or mucosa, including eyes, mouth, esophagus, anus, and vagina can be infected if they come into direct contact, usually transmitted by kissing, sharing plates, glasses, bottles, intercourse with the affected infectious persons. Also touching the affected areas with hands and fingers, and then touching (without washing hands) any other areas, such as eyes, mouth, anus, vagina, can easily infect them. It is very important to wash your hands frequently, particularly before and after applying medication.

Herpes simplex virus type 2 creates painful liquid-filled blisters on the moist linings surrounding the genital organs. Initially, the affected person feels itchy, burning, and tingling sensations surrounding the sex organs, and also mild fever. Some women find a connection between menstrual cycle and herpes outbreak. Acidic foods, such as animal products, including diary products, or excess intake of protein,, highly chemically processed foods, may activate the outbreaks. It is a common belief that the condition of immune deficiency connected to stress, anxiety, and dietary indiscretions can tip the balance in favour of outbreaks.

It is important to note that a pregnant woman infected with herpes simplex virus type 2 may pass on to her baby during natural birth letting the baby form lesions from direct contact, and disorders in its nervous system, such as seizures and mental retardation. Pregnant women should be screened for infection during their pregnancies, and caesarean birth can prevent the transmission of herpes simplex virus type 2 to the baby.

CHAPTER TEN

Treatment

Diet
-   **avoid arginine-rich foods:** chocolates, peanuts, almonds, cashew, pecans, garlic, carob, and wheat. Arginine is an amino acid that may trgger outbreak of herpes.

-   Avoid foods that compromise your immune system: refined sugars, preservatives, processed foods…..etc

-   Identify your personal food sensitivities; (e.g., diary, eggs, wheat, corn, sugar .)

-   Avoid **acidic foods**, such as excessive intake of proteins (specially animal foods), grapefruits, tomatoes, oranges, other citrus fruits. These foods may aggravate cold sores, and should be avoided during an outbreak.

-   Reduce stress through meditation, pranayama, (positive affirmation and visualization Recommended Diet

- consume foods that are rich in the amino acid L-lysine

Conventional Therapy

Traditional treatments include topical and oral antiviral prescription drugs, such as acyclover'

Topical Remedies (or Ointments)
-   L-lysine ointment. Apply topically four times daily or as required

-   Thymus ointment. Apply four times daily or as required

-   Zinc: 0.025 % (topical)

-   Myrrh tincture (topical)

-   Colloidal silver; apply topically

-   Apply topically 3 drops of Melissa, essential oik diluted with ¼ tsp of aloe vera gel three to four times daily

-   Ice (early stages of outbreaks) apply to affected areas for ten or fifteen minutes. Repeat frequently throughout the day. Apply vitamin E in between.

Natural Supplements

Any high potency (at least 50 mg) twice daily) multiple vitamins rich with minerals would normally contain the following ingredients, such as

-   vitamin A, 10,000 – 25000 IU daily

-   vitamin B complex 50 mg 1 – 3 times daily

-   B12, 2000 (2g) twice daily (may be intravenously)

-   Zinc, 25-50 1-2 times daily (age over 14)

-   Selenium 200 mcg twice daily

-   Omega 3-6-9

All these above ingredients can be found in any high potency multiple vitamins rich with minerals.

Next take vitamin C with bioflavonoids, 1000 mg three time daily.

Other Therapeutic Agents

- L-lysine, 1000-2000 mg between meals three times daily if it is acute.

- Consume foods rich in lysine, such as   beans, eggs, brewer's yeast, potatoes, and fish;

- Probiotics; one capsule 3 times daily.

Herbs
- cayenne; stimulates the circulatory system;

- Echinacea; bolsters immune system response;

- Goldenseal roots; (hydrastis Canadensis): 2 capsules or 50 drops of a liquid extract taken twice daily. Also, apply liquid extract directly on the cold sores several times daily. This may help control infection and reduce inflammation;

- Lomatium root (lomatium dissectum): it is a potent antiviral. 2 caps. or 50 drops of liquid extract twice daily;

- Licorice root (glycyrrhiza uralensis or glabra): 2 caps or 50 drops of liquid extract twice daily. It can also be used topically as a gel. The study bt Dr. Melvyn Werbach, MD, University of California, Los Angeles, School of Medicine, noted that a mouth wash containing this herb provided relief for 75 % of the people who used it, got substantial relief within a day, and complete healing in three days;

-

  In addition to to containing tannin, it also contains two compounds---glycyrrhetinic-
  Acid and glycyrrhizin that inhibit the growth of herpes simplex virus. Furthermore,
  They also help speed of the healing of sores.

- myrrh ((commiphora myrrha): myrrh is used for the treatment of inflammation of
  mouth and throat, contains high amounts of tannin (tannic acid), a substance contained in many plants and gives foods an astringent taste. It is antiseptic with a wide-spectrum of anti-bacterial and anti-viral effects, 3especially useful for treating mouth sores, caused by bacteria, fungi, and viruses or allergies;

Doses: 2 capsules or 50 drops of liquid extract twice daily. Also dab liquid extract directly to the affected areas several times daily. This may produce useful astringent and antiviral effects;

- wild geranium (geranium maculatum): this herb also contains high amounts of tannin, used as an astringent to stop bleeding of open wounds and as a wash to treat cold sores;

- St. John's wort: antiviaral, especially against enveloped viruses.

Homeopathy

- Arsenicum: Cold sores, epithelioma of lips, with burning and shooting pain which becomes worse at night. Ulceration of mouth with dryness and burning heat. Crusts are large, and deep, and bleed when peeled.

-

  Doses (6-30 CH, in liquid or pellets): liquid spray under the tongue or as required; if it is in pellets, put six pellets of 6 ch or 3 pellets of 30 ch under the tongue; 3 times daily, or as advised by the health care professional'

- Arsenicum Brom: it has been proven to be a great remedy for anti-psoric, antisyphil-itic, herpetic eruptions, and syphilitic excrescences (swelling outgrowth, eruptions, cancer, boil, carbuncle, pus-filled inflammation) Dose: see instruction above;

- Dulcamara (6-30 ch): cold sores on lips, worse in slightest exposure to cold. Humid uptions on face, genitals, and hands. Thick yellow crusts, bleeding when peeled
  Dose: follow the above instructions

- Hepar Sulph (6-30 ch): cold sores in the middle of the lower lip. Upper lip swollen and tender. Neuralgia of right side extending to temple, ear, and lips. Ulcers in the corner of the mouth. Again for doses see above

- mercurius: cold sore outbreaks accompanied by drooling and fever, fetid odour from mouth, can smell it all over room, worse at night,, on damp, rainy, and cold weather.

  Caution: Most herbal extracts contain alcohol. Avoid using them if you are sensitive to alcohol or you have an history of abuse. However, alcohol content can evaporates if the extract is added to very hot water (close to boiling point) and allowing it to stand for 10 to 15 minutes before drinking.

  Reference
  www.coldsores.net/

GOOD LUCK